Smarter Not Harder: The Guide to Efficient and Effective Living

Cecilia N. Johnson

Table of contents

CHAPTER 1.

Introduction: Working Smarter, Not Harder Explanation of the concept

The concept of working smarter, not harder is based on the idea that achieving success and achieving goals requires more than just putting in hours and hard work. Instead, he emphasizes the importance of strategy, efficiency, and productivity in his work.

Working smarter involves identifying the most important tasks and focusing on them first, and leveraging technology and other tools to automate or streamline repetitive tasks or time consuming. It also involves setting clear priorities, managing time effectively, and constantly looking for ways to improve processes and workflows.

By working smarter, individuals can achieve better results with less effort, reduce stress and burnout, and have more time and energy for other important aspects of their lives. life, such as family, hobbies or personal growth. Ultimately, the goal is to increase productivity and success while maintaining a healthy work-life balance.

The importance of working smarter

Working smarter is important for several reasons:

Effective:By working smarter, you can achieve the same results in less time, using fewer resources. This means you can get more done in a day, which is important if you have a lot of tasks to complete.

Productivity:Working smarter also means you can be more productive. By focusing on the most important tasks and using your time wisely, you can get more done in less time. Best results:

When you work smarter, you can get better results. By focusing on the most important tasks and using your time and resources efficiently, you can achieve better results.

Reduce stress:Working smarter can also help reduce stress. When you can manage your time and tasks effectively, you're less likely to feel overwhelmed or stressed.

Career development:Working smarter can also help advance your career. Employers value employees who are efficient, productive, and able to achieve good results. By working smarter, you can showcase these qualities and increase your chances of career advancement.

Overall, working smarter is essential for success in your personal and professional life. This allows you to work more efficiently, be more productive and achieve better results, while reducing stress and advancing your career.

The benefits of working smarter
Working smarter can have many benefits, including:
Increase productivity:When you work smarter, you can focus on the things that matter most and get them done more efficiently. This can lead to increased productivity and better results in less time.

Improve work-life balance:By working smarter, you can often get more done in less time, which can help you achieve a better balance between work and personal life.

Less pressure:Working smarter can help you avoid feeling overwhelmed or exhausted by your workload. By prioritizing tasks and using effective time management strategies, you can reduce stress and improve your overall health.

Higher job satisfaction:When you can work smarter and achieve your goals more efficiently, you can feel more satisfied and accomplished in your work. Increase creativity:By working smarter, you can free up more mental energy and space to think creatively and find creative solutions to problems.

Overall, working smarter can help you get more done while reducing stress and improving your quality of life.

CHAPTER 2

Assessing Your Current Work Habits

As an AI language model, I don't have the same working habits as a human because I have no physical or emotional needs. However, I can offer some general advice for evaluating and improving work habits.

Track your time:Start by assessing how you are currently spending your time. Use a time tracking app or just write down what you're doing and how long it takes. This will give you a better idea of how you're spending your time and where you might be wasting it. Define your priorities:
Make a list of your goals and priorities, both short and long term. This will help you focus your time and energy on the things that matter most.

Create a schedule:Once you've identified your priorities, create a schedule that allows you to consistently execute them. This could mean spending specific time on certain tasks or spending certain days of the week on specific projects.

Minimize distractions:Identify the t ahhings that distract you the most and find ways to minimize them. That could mean turning off phone or email notifications at certain times of the day, or finding a quiet workspace where you can focus without interruption.

Breaks:Taking regular breaks can actually make you more productive in the long run. Be sure to schedule short breaks during the day to rest and recharge.

Reflect and adjust:Regularly evaluate your progress and adjust your routine as needed. This will keep you on track and improve over time. Remember that everyone's work habits are different, so it's important to figure out what works best for you. By assessing your current habits and making necessary adjustments, you can increase your productivity and achieve your goals more efficiently.

Identifying time-wasting activities can be helpful in increasing productivity and efficiency. Here are some common examples of time-wasting activities:

Social scrolling:Spending too much time on social media platforms, scrolling through news feeds and timelines can be a huge waste of time.

Multitasking:Trying to do too many things at once can reduce productivity and quality of work. The delay: Postponing tasks or putting them off until the last minute can lead to unnecessary stress and time pressure.

Excessive meetings:Attending irrelevant or poorly organized meetings can be a huge waste of time.

Emails and Messages:
Constantly checking and responding to emails, texts, and notifications can be a huge waste of time.

Unnecessary interruption:Frequent interruptions by coworkers, phone calls, or other distractions can hinder productivity and disrupt concentration.

Lack of organization:Not having a clear plan or structure for the day can lead to wasted time and inefficiencies. Identifying these time-consuming activities can help individuals and organizations take steps to reduce them and improve productivity.

Evaluating productivity levels
Evaluating productivity levels can be an important task for individuals, groups and organizations to determine the efficiency and effectiveness of the work performed. Here are a few ways to measure productivity:

Output Measurements:Output measures measure the amount of work produced. This could include the number of products produced, the number of sales generated, or the number of tasks completed within a given time frame.

Input Measurements:Input figures estimate the resources needed to create a job. This could include the number of hours worked, the amount spent, or the number of employees assigned to a project. Quality index:

Quality measures measure the excellence of the work produced. This could include customer satisfaction, the accuracy of completed tasks, or the rate of errors made in the manufacturing process.

Time management:Time management is an important part of productivity as it measures how effectively time is used to get things done. This may include time spent on non-productive activities or the time required to complete a task by a set deadline.

Staff comments:Asking for employee feedback is another way to gauge productivity levels. This may include surveys, interviews, or focus groups to gauge how well employees feel they can get their work done and what barriers they face.

Overall, assessing productivity levels requires a multifaceted approach that considers both quantitative and qualitative factors. By measuring productivity levels, individuals, teams, and organizations can identify areas
  improvement and make adjustments to optimize performance and efficiency.

Assess work-life balance Assessing work-life balance involves assessing how well a person is able to manage and prioritize work and personal responsibilities in a way that allows them to maintain a sense of satisfaction, satisfaction, and satisfaction. common heart and happiness. Here are some factors to consider when assessing work-life balance:

Time spent on work:Time spent at work can be a good indicator of work-life balance. Working long hours and constantly checking work-related emails or texts can negatively impact an individual's personal life.

Personal time:Individuals should have enough time for hobbies, social activities, exercise, and rest. Lack of personal time can lead to burnout and stress.

Flexible:Having flexible working hours or the ability to work from home can help individuals achieve a better work-life balance.

Stress level:High levels of stress can indicate an imbalance between work and personal life. It is important to identify the causes of stress and find ways to manage them effectively.

Relationships:Maintaining healthy relationships with family and friends is important for a good work-life balance. Lack of quality time with loved ones can lead to feelings of isolation and loneliness.

Mental and physical health:Prioritizing physical and mental health is important to overall health. This includes getting enough sleep, eating healthy, participating in regular exercise and self-care activities.

By assessing these factors, individuals can better understand their work-life balance and take steps to improve it if necessary. It's important to remember that work-life balance is unique to each individual and can change over time based on personal and professional circumstances.

Strategies for Working Smarter

Prioritizing tasksPrioritizing tasks is a crucial skill for being productive and achieving your goals. Here are some steps you can take to prioritize your tasks effectively:

Make a list of all the tasks you need to complete. Write them down in a notebook, on a whiteboard, or in a digital tool like Trello or Asana.

Determine the urgency of each task. Which tasks need to be done today or tomorrow? Which ones can wait until next week?

Determine the importance of each task. Which tasks will have the biggest impact on your goals or your work? Which ones are necessary to move your projects forward?
Rank your tasks in order of priority. Use a numbering system, color coding, or any other method that works for you.

Break down larger tasks into smaller, more manageable sub-tasks. This can help you tackle complex projects more efficiently and make progress more quickly.

Be flexible and adjust your priorities as needed. Sometimes unexpected events or urgent tasks will arise, and you may need to reprioritize your to-do list.

By following these steps, you can create a prioritized list of tasks that will help you stay focused and productive throughout the day.

Using time management techniques
Time management is the process of organizing and planning how much time you spend on various tasks in order to maximize productivity and efficiency. Here are some time management techniques that you can use to help manage your time more effectively:

Set goals and prioritize tasks: Start by setting clear goals and identifying the most important tasks that need to be completed. Prioritize your tasks based on their importance and urgency.

Create a schedule: Create a daily or weekly schedule that includes blocks of time for specific tasks. Stick to your schedule as closely as possible to ensure that you are making progress towards your goals.

Use time-tracking tools: Use tools like timers or time-tracking software to help you monitor how much time you spend on each task. This will help you identify areas where you may be wasting time and make adjustments accordingly.

Eliminate distractions: Eliminate distractions by turning off notifications on your phone or computer and finding a quiet workspace. This will help you focus on the task at hand and complete it more efficiently.

Take breaks: Take short breaks between tasks to give your brain a chance to rest and recharge. This will help you stay focused and avoid burnout.

Delegate tasks: If possible, delegate tasks to others who are better suited to complete them. This will free up your time to focus on more important tasks.

Learn to say no: Learn to say no to requests that are not aligned with your goals or priorities. This will help you avoid overcommitting yourself and ensure that you have enough time to complete the tasks that are most important.

By using these time management techniques, you can improve your productivity, reduce stress, and achieve your goals more effectively.

Automating and delegating tasks
Automating and delegating tasks can be a great way to increase productivity and efficiency in your work or

personal life. Here are some tips and considerations for automating and delegating tasks:

Automating Tasks:
Identify repetitive tasks that take a significant amount of time
Research software or tools that can automate these tasks
Evaluate the cost-benefit of implementing the automation, including the time and cost required to set it up and the time and cost savings it will provide in the long run
Test the automation thoroughly before implementing it in your workflow
Monitor the automation regularly to ensure it is working properly and make adjustments as needed

Delegating Tasks:

Identify tasks that can be delegated to others, such as tasks that are outside of your expertise or tasks that are not a good use of your time
Consider the skills and availability of the people you can delegate tasks to
Clean Automating and delegating tasks
Automating and delegating tasks can be a great way to increase productivity and efficiency in your work or personal life. Here are some tips and considerations for automating and delegating tasks:

Automating Tasks:

Identify repetitive tasks that take a significant amount of time

Research software or tools that can automate these tasks

Evaluate the cost-benefit of implementing the automation, including the time and cost required to set it up and the time and cost savings it will provide in the long run

Test the automation thoroughly before implementing it in your workflow

Monitor the automation regularly to ensure it is working properly and make adjustments as needed

Delegating Tasks:

Identify tasks that can be delegated to others, such as tasks that are outside of your expertise or tasks that are not a good use of your time

Consider the skills and availability of the people you can delegate tasks to

Communicate the expectations and requirements for the task, including deadlines and any specific instructions

Provide the necessary resources and support for the person you are delegating the task to, such as training or access to information

Follow up regularly to ensure the task is on track and provide feedback or adjustments as needed

Remember that both automation and delegation require some upfront investment of time and effort, but can lead to significant time and cost savings in the long run.

Taking breaks and avoiding burnout

Taking breaks and avoiding burnout is crucial for maintaining productivity and overall well-being. Here are some tips to help you take breaks and avoid burnout:

Schedule regular breaks:Schedule regular breaks throughout your day to allow your mind and body to rest and recharge. This can be as simple as taking a 10-minute walk, having a snack, or doing some stretching exercises. Focus on personal care:

Make self-care a priority in your daily routine. This can include getting enough sleep, eating healthy, exercising regularly, and spending time engaging in activities that bring you joy and relaxation.

Take a vacation: Plan regular vacations or time off from work to allow yourself to disconnect and recharge. Even a short break can help you come back to work feeling refreshed and re-energized.

Remember, taking care of yourself is important for your mental and physical health, and it will ultimately help you be more productive and successful in the long run.

CHAPTER 3:

Developing a Productive Mindset

Developing an effective mindset is essential to achieving your goals and progressing in your personal and professional life. Here are some strategies that can help you cultivate effective thinking:

Set yourself clear goals:Having clear goals keeps you focused and motivated. Write down your goals and break them down into smaller, achievable steps.

Task Priority:Prioritize tasks that help you make the most of your time and energy. Identify the most important tasks and complete them first. Focus on solutions:
Instead of focusing on problems, focus on finding solutions. Be proactive and find ways to overcome obstacles.
Complete the challenge:Challenges are opportunities to grow and learn. Accept them and see them as opportunities for self-improvement.
Manage your time wisely:Time is a precious resource, so use it wisely. Set deadlines for tasks and avoid procrastination.

Maintain a positive attitude:A positive attitude helps you stay motivated and focused. Be optimistic and focus on the positive aspects of your work.

Breaks:Taking breaks helps you recharge and avoid burnout. Schedule regular breaks and use them to do something you enjoy. Take care :
Taking care of your physical and mental health is essential to productivity. Eat right, exercise, get enough sleep, and take care of your mental health.

By applying these strategies, you can cultivate productive thinking and achieve your goals more easily and effectively.

Adopt a growth mindset Adopting a growth mindset means accepting the idea that your abilities and intelligence can be developed through dedication and hard work. This is in contrast to a fixed mindset, where you believe your abilities and intelligence are predetermined and cannot be changed. To adopt a growth mindset, you can start by:
Join the challenge:Instead of avoiding challenges and sticking with what you're comfortable with, embrace new challenges and see them as opportunities to learn and grow.
Persevere to overcome obstacles:Don't give up easily in the face of setbacks or setbacks. Instead, see them as opportunities to learn and try again.

Make an effort:Realize that effort and hard work are essential for growth and improvement. Instead of relying on your innate talent or intelligence, focus on constantly striving to improve yourself. Search reviews:
Instead of avoiding comments or criticism, actively seek them out and use them as an opportunity to learn and grow.
Learn from others:Realize that you can learn from others and seek out mentors or role models who can inspire and teach you.

By adopting a growth mindset, you can develop a passion for learning and improving, which can help you be more successful in all areas of your life.

Developing positive habits Developing positive habits can be difficult, but with a little dedication and commitment, it is completely doable. Here are some tips to help you develop positive habits:

Small start:Don't try to change everything at once. Focus on one or two habits you want to develop at a time. This will keep you from feeling overwhelmed and increase your chances of success.

Be specific:Clearly define the habit you want to develop. For example, instead of saying "I want to exercise more", say "I want to exercise 30 minutes a day".

Determine the target:Set specific, achievable goals for your routine. It will give you something to work with and keep you motivated. Create a routine:
Develop a routine or schedule that includes your routine. For example, if you want to read more, set aside a specific time each day to read.

Track your progress:Track your progress so you can see how far you've come. This will help keep you motivated and on track.

Celebrate your successes:Celebrate your success, no matter how small
it may seem. It will help you stay positive and

Stay accountable: Share your goals and progress with a friend or family member. Having someone to hold you accountable can be a powerful motivator.

Remember, developing positive habits takes time and effort. But with some dedication and commitment, you can create lasting change in your life.

Overcoming procrastination
Procrastination is a common problem that affects many people and it can be difficult to break the habit. However, there are a few strategies you can use to overcome procrastination:
Break down tasks into smaller, more manageable chunks. Big tasks can be overwhelming and easy to

procrastinate. By breaking a task into smaller chunks, you can make it more manageable and less daunting.

Set specific and achievable goals. Instead of setting vague goals, set yourself specific and achievable goals. This will keep you focused and motivated, and you can measure your progress.

Create a schedule or to-do list. Having a schedule or to-do list can help you stay organized and prioritize your tasks. It can also help you avoid distractions and focus on your tasks. Eliminate distractions. Distractions can be a big obstacle to getting things done. Try to eliminate distractions as much as possible. This could mean turning off your phone, closing unnecessary tabs on your computer, or finding a quiet place to work.

Use the Pomodoro technique. The Pomodoro Technique is a time management strategy that involves working for a set amount of time (usually 25 minutes) and taking short breaks. It can help you focus and avoid burnout.

Hold yourself accountable. It can be helpful to have someone hold you accountable for completing a task. It could be a friend, family member or co-worker. You can also use an app or website that tracks your progress and sends you reminders.

Remember, overcoming procrastination takes time and effort. It's important to be patient with yourself and keep trying different strategies until you find the one that works best for you.

Stay motivated and focused Staying motivated and focused can be difficult at times, but there are several strategies you can use to help you stay focused and motivated:

Set clear goals:Define what you want to achieve and break your goals down into smaller, achievable tasks. This will help you stay focused and motivated as you work towards your goals. Create a routine:

Establish a consistent routine that includes regular exercise, healthy eating, and adequate sleep. It will keep you energized and focused throughout the day.

Remove distractions:Identify and eliminate any distractions that might be hindering your productivity, such as social media, email notifications, or other interruptions. Consider using productivity tools or apps to help you focus.

Increased optimism:Cultivate a positive mindset by focusing on your strengths, celebrating your successes, and learning from your mistakes. Surround yourself with positive, supportive people who can help keep you motivated.

Breaks:Give yourself regular breaks during the day to rest and recharge. Short breaks can help improve your focus and productivity when you get back to work.

Visualize success:Imagine that you achieve your goal and will get a positive result. Visualizing success can help you stay focused and on track to achieve your goals. Remember that staying motivated and focused is an ongoing process that requires commitment and effort. With consistent practice and the right mindset, you can develop the habits and strategies you need to achieve your goals, while staying motivated and focused along the way.

CHAPTER 4:

Improve communication and collaboration

Improved communication and collaboration can dramatically improve the efficiency and productivity of teams, whether working in a physical or remote office. Here are some tips to improve communication and collaboration in teams:

Set up clear communication channels:It's important to establish clear channels of communication within your team, whether through email, messaging apps, video conferencing, or project management tools. Make sure everyone knows how to use these channels effectively, and establish guidelines for when and how to use them.

Encourage open communication:
Encourage your team members to share their ideas, concerns, and feedback openly and honestly. Create a safe and inclusive environment where people feel comfortable expressing themselves. Practice active listening:
When someone speaks, listen actively and attentively. This means paying attention to what the person is

saying, asking clarifying questions, and reflecting on what you've heard to make sure you got it right.

Set up regular subscriptions:Regular check-ins can help ensure everyone is on the same page and that any issues or concerns are addressed quickly. Schedule weekly or biweekly team meetings to discuss progress, goals, and challenges.

Use collaboration tools:Collaboration tools like shared documents, project management software, and task boards can help teams stay organized, track progress, and collaborate more effectively. Nurturing a culture of cooperation:
Encourage your team members to work together and support each other. Foster a culture of collaboration and teamwork by recognizing and celebrating individual and team achievements.

Provide constructive feedback:Provide constructive feedback to your team members to help them improve and grow. Make sure your feedback is specific, actionable, and sent in a positive way.
By implementing these tips, you can improve communication and collaboration in your team and achieve better results. Effective communication techniques

Effective communication is an essential skill in personal and professional contexts. Here are some techniques for effective communication:

Active listening:Listen attentively to the person who is speaking and show that you are listening by nodding or using affirmative words.

Clarify:If you don't understand what the person is saying, ask questions to clarify.

Empathetic:Try to understand the other person's point of view and use empathy to build rapport and trust.

Be clear and concise:Use clear and simple language, avoid jargon or technical jargon, and keep your message short. Non-verbal communication:
Pay attention to nonverbal cues such as facial expressions, body language, and tone of voice to gauge the speaker's feelings and intentions.

Respect:Show respect for the ideas and opinions of others, even if you disagree with them.

Comment:Provide constructive feedback and be open to receiving feedback from others.
hourly:Choose the right time and place to send your message, taking into account the other person's schedule and mood.

Adapt to the audience:Tailor your communication style and message to the needs and preferences of your audience. Follow up:

Follow up after the conversation to make sure both sides are on the same page and to address any remaining concerns.

Collaboration with team members is an essential part of the success of any project or task. Here are some tips to help you collaborate effectively with your team:
Communicate:Communication is key when it comes to collaboration. Make sure to establish clear lines of communication and keep everyone on the same page throughout the project.

Define roles and responsibilities:Make sure all team members understand their roles and responsibilities. This will ensure that everyone knows what is expected of them and can work together more effectively.
Set goals and deadlines:Set clear goals and timelines for the project. This will keep everyone focused and motivated, and will ensure the project stays on track.

Use collaboration tools:There are many collaboration tools available, such as project management software,

CHAPTER 5:

Leveraging Technology for Efficiency

Leveraging technology for efficiency can bring enormous benefits to businesses and individuals. Here are a few ways to do that:

Automate tasks: Many tasks can be automated with technology, such as scheduling appointments, sending emails, and updating spreadsheets. This frees up time for more important tasks and reduces the risk of mistakes.

Use collaboration tools: Collaboration tools like project management software, video conferencing, and cloud storage can help teams work together more efficiently. These tools can streamline communication, document sharing, and project tracking. Set up a digital filing system:
Storing documents electronically can save time and space. It also facilitates the search and retrieval of documents. Consider using a cloud-based document management system.

Using mobile technology: Mobile devices can provide access to important information on the go and enable employees to work remotely. This can increase productivity and flexibility. Apply artificial intelligence:
AI can help automate repetitive tasks, provide insights from data, and even make predictions. Consider implementing a chatbot, virtual assistant, or AI-powered predictive analytics software.

By leveraging technology in these ways, individuals and businesses can increase efficiency, reduce costs, and improve productivity. However, it is important to also consider potential risks and downsides, such as privacy and data security issues.

Use productivity tools and apps Productivity tools and apps are software designed to help you be more productive. These tools can be used to manage tasks, schedule meetings, organize notes, collaborate with colleagues, and more. Here are some tips for using productivity tools and apps effectively:

Choose the right tools:There are many productivity tools and apps available, so it's important to choose the ones and apps that best suit your needs. Consider your working style, the tasks you need to perform, and the features that are important to you when choosing your tool.

Check out the features:Take the time to explore the features of your productivity tools and apps. Many programs have hidden features or shortcuts that can save you time and increase productivity. Integration with other tools:

Many productivity tools and applications can be integrated with other software. For example, you can link the calendar app to the mail app to easily schedule meetings.

Set reminder:Use reminders to help you stay on track and complete tasks on time. Set reminders for deadlines, meetings, and other important events.

Task Priority:Use your productivity tools and apps to prioritize tasks based on importance and urgency. It can help you focus on the most important tasks and ensure they are completed on time.

Collaborate with others:There are many productivity tools and apps available to collaborate with others. Use these features to work more efficiently with your colleagues and teammates.

Using the mobile app:Many productivity tools and apps have mobile apps that let you access them on the go. Use these apps to stay productive even when you're away from your desk. Overall, using productivity tools and apps can help you be more productive. By choosing the right tools, learning their features, and using them effectively, you can increase your productivity and achieve your goals faster.

Automate and streamline processes

Process automation and streamlining refer to the use of technologies and systematic approaches to optimize and simplify business operations. This involves identifying areas that can be automated and using technology to reduce or eliminate manual tasks, thereby

improving efficiency, reducing costs, and increasing productivity.

Process automation involves using software or tools to automate repetitive tasks that were previously performed manually, such as data entry, invoicing, and customer service... By automating these tasks, businesses can save time and resources and focus on more important activities.

Building a Support System Building a support system is key to maintaining good mental and emotional health. Having people around you who can give you emotional support, guidance, and help you through tough times can make a huge difference in your happiness. Here are some tips for creating a support system:

Identify the people in your life who are supportive and trustworthy. This could be a family member, friend, co-worker, or therapist.

Reach out to these people and let them know you appreciate their support. This could involve chatting with them, texting them, or just spending more time with them.

Be open and honest with your support system about your feelings and difficulties. It's important to communicate what you need, whether it's a listening ear, a hug, or practical help.

Nurture new relationships and connections. Consider joining a support group, volunteering, or participating in social activities to meet new people who share your interests and values. Take care of yourself and seek professional help if needed. Building a support system is an important step, but it's also important that you take care of yourself and ask for help when you need it. This may involve seeking the advice of a mental health professional or practicing self-care techniques such as meditation or exercise.

Remember that building a support system takes time and effort, but it's worth it because of the benefits it can bring. Having a network of supporters can help you face life's challenges with greater resilience and confidence. Surround yourself with positivity
affect
Surrounding yourself with positive influences can have a significant impact on your overall happiness and success in life. Positive influences can take many forms, such as supportive friends and family members, motivational speakers, mentors, role models, or even positive media content.

Having positive people around you can boost your self-esteem, boost your motivation, and help you maintain a positive outlook on life. These people can give you emotional support, guidance and advice during difficult times, and can help you see the best in yourself and others.

On the contrary, negative influences can drag you down, frustrate you and drain your energy. Negative influences can include toxic people, pessimistic attitudes, and destructive behavior. These people can create stress, anxiety, and feelings of hopelessness, which can harm your mental and physical health.

Therefore, it is important to evaluate the people and things around you and make conscious choices to surround you with positive influences. This may involve making new friends, finding new hobbies or activities that inspire you, and avoiding situations or people that drain you of energy or bring you down.

By surrounding yourself with positive influences, you can create a supportive and uplifting environment that helps you achieve your goals and live life to the fullest.
Build relationships with mentors and peers
Building relationships with mentors and peers is important for personal and professional growth. Here are some tips for building those relationships:

Verified:Authenticity is key when it comes to building relationships with mentors and peers. Be yourself and let your personality shine through.

Be respected:Treat your mentors and colleagues with respect. Consider their time and expertise. Show interest:
Show interest in their work and ask questions. This will show your curiosity and desire to learn.

Active listening:Actively listen to what your mentors and peers have to say. Pay attention to their ideas and suggestions.

Clear communication:Communicate clearly and effectively. Be sure to express yourself in an understandable way.

Reliable:Be trustworthy and keep your commitments. This will demonstrate your credibility and commitment.

Unified:Support your mentors and colleagues. Help and encourage when they ,

Seeking help when needed It is important to recognize when you need help and to seek it out when necessary. Asking for help can be difficult for some people, but it is a sign of strength and courage to reach out for support when needed. Here are some tips for seeking help:

Identify the problem: First, identify the specific problem you are facing. This will help you communicate your needs more effectively when seeking help.

Decide who to ask: Think about who is best suited to help you with your particular issue. It might be a friend, family member, teacher, or professional.

Be clear and specific: When asking for help, be clear and specific about what you need. This will help the person you are asking to understand your situation and provide you with the best support.

Be open to feedback: Be open to feedback and suggestions from others. They may have insights or ideas that you have not considered before.

Express gratitude: Finally, remember to express gratitude to the person who helped you. Whether it is a simple thank you or a kind gesture, showing appreciation for their help can go a long way in building positive relationships.

CHAPTER 6:

Conclusion: Working Smarter for Long-Term Success

Working smart, not hard, is the key to long-term success in your personal and professional life. Focus on what matters most, prioritize goals, and maximize efficiency and productivity.

To work smarter, you need to have a clear understanding of your goals and break them down into smaller achievable goals. This allows you to focus your time and energy on the most important tasks that will have the greatest impact on your success.

It is also important to develop good habits and habits such as: B. Schedule time for focused work, take breaks to recharge, and maintain a healthy work-life balance. In this way, burnout can be prevented and motivation and performance maintained over the long term.

In addition, seeking learning and development opportunities through formal education and on-the-job training will help you continuously improve your skills and keep abreast of industry trends.

Overall, working smarter means working consciously and strategically, continuously looking for ways to improve and optimize performance. This will allow you to have more success and fulfillment in all areas of your life.

Summary strategies and techniques Encouragement to keep working smarter

safety! Here's an overview of some strategies and techniques to help you work smarter.

Prioritize your tasks:Prioritize tasks based on urgency and importance. This helps you focus on your most important tasks first and complete them on time.

Categorize your tasks.Break down large tasks into smaller, more manageable tasks. This way you can avoid feeling overwhelmed and work on your projects more easily.

Use productivity tools.Stay organized and manage your time more effectively with productivity tools like task managers, calendars, and time tracking software.

Block of time:Time blocking is the technique of assigning specific time slots to tasks and activities. This will help you stay on course and avoid distractions.

Get a break:Taking breaks actually helps you be more productive. Taking a break gives your brain a chance to rest and recharge.

Agent:If you have tasks that can be delegated, consider delegating them. Delegating tasks can buy you time to focus on more important tasks. learn to say no
It can be hard to say no, but it's important to prioritize your time and only take on tasks that align with your goals and priorities.

Remember that working smarter takes time and effort. You can feel the benefits in your work and private life. Good luck!

Final Thoughts and Advice.on Smarter not hard

"Work smarter, not harder" is a famous saying that emphasizes the importance of finding efficient and effective ways to get things done. Here are some final thoughts and advice on how to work smarter and work harder.
Prioritize your tasks:Identify your most important tasks and focus your energy and resources on completing them first. This will increase your productivity and give you better results.

Automate repetitive tasks:We use technology and tools to automate repetitive tasks so you can focus on more important and complex tasks.

Get a break:Taking regular breaks can actually help you be more productive by preventing burnout and recharging your batteries.

Learn new skills:Continuous learning and development helps you improve your skills and find more efficient ways to get things done.

Collaborate with others:Working with others can bring new perspectives and ideas to help you achieve your goals more efficiently. Plan your day:

Plan your day ahead and set specific goals for what you want to achieve. This will keep you on track